NONTOXIC
Teeth Whitening
and
Dental Hygiene
SYSYEM

Chapters 9 & 10 taken from the
NCD Flaxseed Shake Recipe
(not included – available online)

Chapters 11 & 12 (New)
Food Grade & JPM Whitening™

Chapters 13 & 14 (New)
Commentary on Fluoride

Free Report – JPM Nontoxic Hand Sanitizer™

Jumper Publications and Media

Other Publications

ABC Water and the Number Crunch Diet
a step by step solution to alkaline deficiency and
with a New and Unique approach to weight control

JPM Oral Hygiene Protocol
stop using toxic drugstore mouthwash, discover how to reduce
your gum pocket depth from 3-4-3 to 1-2-1 mm when they probe

NCD Flaxseed Shake Recipe
the Number Crunch Diet method for getting omega 3s
and with three variations so you'll never get bored

12 Changes A Year – Volume 1
the recipe book to the Number Crunch Diet
When you take control of the numbers
you take control of your weight.

The 5 Points of Posture
the missing link to fat loss, overall wellness, and
to becoming Respected, Adored, and Wealthy

12 Changes A Year – Volume 2
the recipe book to the Number Crunch Diet
Begin today and forever be in control of the numbers you're eating.

Vision Is Possible
Improve your vision and get a facelift for free!
an original vision program targeting your Eye Lids

Au milieu

Hi and Welcome!

If my French is correct, that expression means "midway" or "in the middle of", which is where this starts. This publication was originally published within the *Number Crunch Diet Flaxseed Shake Recipe*, included as a free report at the end of the booklet. Then I extracted it to make it a stand-alone report. And now it's its own booklet.

To go back and redo it changes the timeline of things and just makes it disjointed. So, I prefer to "amend". I think the Founding Fathers would agree with me that it's the best way to expand on something.

So we begin with Chapter 9. If you are looking for a good read, jam-packed with original content, the *NCD Flaxseed Shake Recipe* is 46 pages and would make a good next step. However, just understand that the Number Crunch Diet initial pages, along with the alkalinity component, are found in the main book – *ABC Water and the Number Crunch Diet*.

Enjoy the next six chapters and I'll see you at the end!

CONTENTS

Edits & Format

You will notice oddities in punctuation, spelling, syntax, and perhaps even semantics, within this book. Feel free to let me know, but some of it is done for brevity or to shift emphasis. I use capitals where I see fit, to grab your attention and make it stand out, and I also remove capitals when I don't think they are deserving of them, or to remove emphasis after first usage, i.e., Pyrex becomes pyrex. And french bread, brussels sprouts, and english cucumbers, are spelled lowercase, as we are not going to "link" a European vacation to our food and eating.

Secondly, I will unhyphenate to create rhythm. Grammatically, two or more words that function as an adjective before a noun are supposed to be hyphenated. That's fine. A million-dollar smile, is the adjective "million-dollar" describing the smile. However, this can get redundant after a while, 1&2 3, 1&2 3, 1&2 3. The noun gets all the attention. But what if you want the adjectives to have the emphasis? After all, the adjectives are the descriptive words. So, I will drop the hyphens to allow the adjectives equal emphasis, and to change the pace of the sentence a bit. So if there are no hyphens, read it slower and evenly, one two three four five six seven. A "step-by-step solution" sounds a bit skippy and simplistic, whereas, a "step by step solution" is said slower and sounds more methodical. Hyphenating two words, or joining two words as a compound word, reduces their individual meanings.

With regard to fastfood, healthfood, and seasalt, it's time for these words to evolve into compound words, so the trend starts here.

There are also some fragmented sentences, subject-verb disagreements, and singular/plural violations. When "correcting" certain of these sentences, they lost their emphasis and punch, so I kept them as is.

In the past I've been guilty of judging other author's sentences, only to reread it with the commas, pauses, and then it made perfect sense. So, if there's a comma, then pause, as you may not get to pause later in the sentence. If there's no comma, then don't pause and read it all as one.

I pose questions, but without question marks. Some are rhetorical, but some are to make you Ponder. Great word. Ponder. If you see a question mark at the end, then it requires an answer. If there's no question mark, then you can just say, yeah, no, or hm.

English continues to change, people using it, customize the language to fit what they want to communicate, emphasize, and to make their point from various angles. It also has to have a variety of melodies and rhythms to keep it from being boring. If you find yourself having to reread a sentence, it may be that it's structured that way for that very reason. So take your time. Don't rush. Let the words digest, so that you absorb the material, and hopefully take some of it and make it a part of your life.

Lastly, you will notice that I customized the headers of every page! This is not something Microsoft Word Starter allows you to do. You can only customize three pages, first, even, and odd. So, to get around this I had to create a Page Break every three pages, and as a result, the last line of some of the pages doesn't "justify" to the edge. So I hope that flipping through the upper corners of the pages will assist you in finding the chapter that you are looking for.

You won't see any citations from scientific studies or PubMed, because at JPM we look to a higher source for our reference.

God Bless!

Enjoy the Journey

Email me if you have a question, or if you just want to comment. Your purchase comes with 6-months free support and photos.

Barry Ogston, B.Sc., CLS, MLS(ASCP)

You have to crunch the numbers to see what you're really eating.

CHAPTER 9

JPM Mouth Rinse Protocol™

In the highly competitive world of publishing and creating a following, a reader base, you've always got to give your audience something for free. This way, if the book was not quite what they thought it was worth, the "free" item will hopefully make up for it. Keep in mind, I price things according to what I would pay for them and according to other things. People pay $250 to see a sporting event, but squawk about the price of information that can positively affect their health for decades to come. A one-night stay in your average hotel room while on vacation can cost $179, and it's long gone. Someone told me he sold a used fishing lure on eBay for $400. What's really going to help you on your journey?

As a lifetime seeker of self-improvement, I have never thought twice about the price if I knew it would benefit me. I left Timothy Ferris, author of *The Four Hour Body*, a 5-star review, even though I had to read all 572 pages of his book to get two things out of it. But, it's two things that I didn't have before I read the book. A person with a lot of these Gold Nuggets is miles ahead in the game of life than someone who just goes along never seeking information. So, there's your good advice. And if you are curious to know what those two things are that I got from his book, stay tuned!

Okay, I'll tell you.

This may not be new to some of you but it was to me.
1. Glut Ham Raises – totally works the backs of your legs.

Not just the hamstrings but the calves and butt as well. Attempt to do 12-15 slow reps in 60 seconds and you will feel it the next day. Best bang for your Back-Of-The-Leg buck. However, for erectors, inner hip muscles, I still like single leg "rocking" deadlifts.

2. MED – Minimal Effective Dose

It's best explained like this. Water comes to a boil when it reaches 100 degrees celsius. Adding more heat, more energy, doesn't make it boil more. Applying this to exercise, it's the old "Stimulate Don't Annihilate" rule. Do one set to failure and that's it. Stop. You're done. Let your muscles break down and regrow bigger. It works. And the best part is, you keep cortisol levels under control. Heavy workouts can zap your body for days, especially when you're over 50!

So this is why *ABC Water and the Number Crunch Diet* is priced like a BMW. It's Revelation Information. A synergy of dozens of books and specialties, to create a completely new book. Selfcare.

So your free report is about "How To Improve Your Gums And Teeth". Two words. Hydrogen Peroxide.

But not so fast. There's the detail.

JPM Mouth Rinse Protocol™

I have to give credit to my brother for this one. He is 62, has never had a cavity, and 33-years ago his dentist told him that he doesn't need to keep coming to the dentist, that, "You're your own dentist."

Now, how many people do you know of that have been told by their dentist that their personal dental hygiene is so good that they are their own dentist and that the dentist actually tells them to stop coming to the dentist? I only know of one. My brother. And he has fantastic teeth and gums, and he's 62, retirement age. What was his secret weapon all these years. Hydrogen Peroxide.

I recall a coworker telling me she had so many dental problems and she was so upset about them. I told her to rinse with hydrogen peroxide. She came back the next week with a big smile on her face, all that anxiety that she had was gone, and she sincerely thanked me profusely. She was smiling bigger and I could tell her gums were looking better already.

Lack of Attached Gingiva. Nobody wants to hear their dentist or dental hygienist say this. Gingiva just means gums. Lack of attached gums, means you have pockets. You know, like when they do the probing of your gums, 334 333 233 432. They go around your teeth checking the pockets of your gums at three locations on each tooth, cheek side and tongue side. Bleeding and pockets means GINGIVITIS. Gum Disease. Bad News.

But there's hope. You can, in my experience, and obviously in my brother's experience, have healthy gums by rinsing with hydrogen peroxide. But there's some do's and don'ts, so keep reading.

I will give you the whole protocol that I do so that you can set it up for yourself at home and begin today to drop those pocket measurements from four and three millimeters to two and one millimeters, and yes, it is possible to have zero mm pockets. Zero mm pockets means you have 100% fully-attached gums to your teeth. My brother has this. You can tell when he smiles. He's got solid gums that are gripped solidly on to his teeth. No pockets. No recession. No Lack of Attached Gingiva.

Of course we have all asked him where he got the idea to rinse with hydrogen peroxide. His answer is brilliant.

"I just thought, well, I'll rinse with hydrogen peroxide."

You see, you don't have to be a doctor to know things, or a PhD, or a licensed blah blah blah. My brother is none of those things. Yet he's a genius when it comes to oral hygiene. AND, the most notable part of his discovery is, It Just Came To Him. Like a thought. Or a revelation. He already had a million-dollar smile, so he was thinking about how he could maintain it and improve on it so that he could have that million dollar big teeth square jaw smile for his whole life.

Imagine having perfect teeth and gums and you haven't been to the dentist in 33 years. In the ABC NCD book I talk about not paying too much attention to crossover double-blind placebo-controlled scientific studies. For some things, the obvious answer is right in front of your face. Just look and believe it. I don't need a study to prove to me that hydrogen-peroxide rinsing can transform bad gum tissue into healthy gum tissue and reduce pocket depth. I use it and it does it. Every one of our family members uses it. We are all following my brother's oral hygiene protocol.

So, here's what you do.

Initial Setup. Buy 8 bottles of 15oz Lea & Perrins Worcestershire sauce at the supermarket. Transfer the liquid to a one-gallon container, or discard it, then proceed to thoroughly rinse the bottles and scrub off the labels. Now you have eight 15oz glass amber bottles with tight-fitting screw caps. The amber color will prevent light from degrading the H_2O_2 into water, and the screw cap will prevent oxygen from getting inside and reacting with the H_2O_2 and converting it into water. So your hydrogen peroxide will stay potent. Also, if you haven't already read my website, we here at JPM and ABC NCD are Plastiphobes. We avoid plastics for eating and for anything that will go in our mouth or used on our body. The HUGE one is, never microwave food in a plastic container, and the lesser evils are, storing the shampoo you use on your head in a plastic container. Replace the plastic containers in your kitchen and bathroom with glass wherever possible.

So, this 15oz bottle is ideal and you'll see why as we go along.

Next. Buy a gallon of hydrogen peroxide. I get mine at Smart & Final supermarket and restaurant-supply store, $8. It's the most economical, $1 per 16oz. And a gallon will keep you from running out. Fill your eight worcester bottles full to the top, to the brim, and then cap them. The bottle holds 16oz exactly, so you have the exact amount needed to fill all 8 bottles to the top. If the bottles were really only 15oz, then 8x15=120oz, and a gallon is 128oz, so you would have 8oz left over. BUT, lucky for you, I have already figured out the perfect bottle.

The other reason for using this bottle is because it has a small mouth. You want to be able to control the amount of hydrogen peroxide entering your mouth as you take a "swig". A wide-mouth bottle will have you pouring in too much H_2O_2 into your mouth. This is important because:

1. Hydrogen peroxide is for external use only. Don't Drink it.
2. If you get too much in your mouth, and it makes contact with the back of your throat, your throat will dry out and you'll end up with a raspy voice.

That brings us to the Technique.
Pucker your lips and use your tongue to control the liquid as it enters your mouth.   When you have about a tablespoon of hydrogen peroxide in your mouth, half an ounce, close your lips and use your cheeks to swirl the liquid around your teeth and gums.

DON'T LET IT TOUCH THE BACK OF YOUR MOUTH

You will have a raspy voice and dry throat if you do.

H_2O_2 IS NOT FOR GARGLING

I will tell you what to use for oral gargling at the end. Your Second Free Report!

So with the H_2O_2 in your mouth, swirl for 30 seconds minimum or 60 seconds maximum. Any less than 30s and you're not doing it long enough for cleaning action to occur, and any longer than 60s and it's no longer doing anything because it's all deactivated, reacted.

Until you get comfortable with this technique, keep your chin down. The natural reaction is to gargle as you are swirling. Don't.

KEEP YOUR CHIN DOWN in the beginning. After a month, the habit should be solidified and you will be able to keep your head in its natural upright position and multitask or stare at yourself in the mirror as you swirl. Are you looking HYA??

Place one of your worcester 16oz hydrogen-peroxide bottles in the shower for your morning oral-hygiene routine, and place the other in the medicine cabinet above your bathroom sink for your before-bed oral-hygiene routine.

16oz will last about one month, 1T, or half an ounce, times 30 days. So, once a month you will start a new bottle in the shower and a new bottle in the medicine cabinet. This is why eight bottles and the one gallon of hydrogen peroxide is the way to do it. When you run out, you just grab another bottle. Two bottles a month means that your eight bottles will last you four months. So every 4 months, or 16 weeks, 3 times a year, you have to pick up a gallon of H_2O_2 and aliquot it into your eight bottles. This is your system.

I gave a bottle to a friend and he freaked out because his gums were foaming up. I said, "Yeah, your gums are foaming up because your gum lines are dirty." He did it twice a day and on the third day they just foamed up a small normal amount. He thanked me profusely.

And I do mean profusely. People are amazed at how amazing this works for reversing bad gums and for making them look that healthy pink color. And no more sensitive areas after a while.

And I've NEVER heard this anywhere. I honestly believe that when this goes viral, mainstream, because of its effectiveness, that the originator was my brother, back in the 1970s, when something, God maybe, inner Divine Intelligence maybe, said, "I think I'll try rinsing with hydrogen peroxide."

You heard it here first. But the credit goes to my brother Ken!

CHAPTER 10

JPM Mouth Wash Protocol™

This next one, I will take credit for. And that's the mouth rinse for gargling, aka, mouth wash.

You know, I've never liked using mouthwash. Whenever I tried it, you know, the typical brand they advertise on TV that starts with the letter L, my eyes would get red and my mouth would burn and I'd spit it out and ask myself.

"Why does mouthwash have to feel so toxic?"

Well, fast-forward to the modern world and we now know that IT IS TOXIC. It's loaded with toxic cancer causing birth defect inducing hormone disrupting CHEMICALS!

You will never convince me that thymol, eucalyptol, methyl salicylate, menthol, alcohol, benzoic acid, poloxamer 407, and caramel, are safe and essential for oral hygiene. Salicylate is aspirin. Why does mouthwash need aspirin? To calm the inflammatory effect from all the chemicals.

And that "alcohol", well, it doesn't say if it's ethanol, the drinkable one, but it could be isopropyl alcohol, rubbing alcohol, the poisonous one, or it could be a mixture of the two. Dr. Hulda Clark in her book, *The Cure For All Diseases*, states that she detects isopropyl alcohol contamination everywhere in our lives because the food industry uses it to sanitize. So the next morning they start up the food-processing machines and all that isopropyl alcohol residue ends up in the food. In trace amounts and randomly, yes, but when you are getting exposed to it from every angle, it begins to build up in the body. She stated in her book that every single cancer patient is toxic with isopropyl alcohol.

There's a group of people who bash her books, and I am not saying she was 100% spot-on with every word she wrote, no person is, and she often said when interviewed that, "We haven't discovered that part yet." But her 604-page book is packed with information and it's the reason that today you hear about pollutants, contamination, chemicals, toxins, detox, and purity. I highlighted and underlined more than half of the book and it took me six months to read it.

So although I take credit for this mouthwash, I really need to give credit to the late Dr. Hulda Clark and *The Cure For All Diseases*. You see, vodka is food-grade alcohol. It's the only food-grade alcohol. And alcohol is a good germ-killer, sanitizer, cleaner, and antiseptic.

JPM Mouth Wash Protocol™

Buy a 1.75 liter bottle of vodka, 40% alcohol by volume, not 25%.

I used to buy the Heritage brand 1.75L 40% vodka at Albertson's supermarket for $9.99, $8.99 on sale, plus tax, but the bottle is plastic.

Plastiphobe

So now I buy the "UV" brand 40% vodka in the 1.75L glass bottle. It's $16.99 at Albertson's, but other grocery stores stock it as well.

I spent a while deciding which glass bottle of vodka to go with, and the UV brand won, as the glass is clear, the shape is smooth, and it has indentations at the back for your hand to grip it. Nice.

40% is too strong for gargling so you will want to dilute it 50/50 half-and-half with water. Go to the healthfood store and buy a few bottles of bottled water in glass. Drink the water and remove the labels. I use Voss brand 400mL cylindrical glass water bottles with screw caps. Nice and classy looking when you get the label cleaned off. Place the bottle on your scale and turn it on. Add 200 grams of vodka, then add 200 grams of water. Voila, 20% vodka.

This is your mouthwash for gargling.

As with the worcester bottles, buy eight Voss water bottles so that you have some ready-to-use when you run out. I use this 20% alcohol to rinse my mouth after meals during the day, along with flossing and brushing. For toothpaste I use Trader Joe's/Tom's brand, with Fennel, Propolis and Myrrh, lavender color on the box.

Tom's brand has been around for a long time and back in the 1980s is was the only Health Food toothpaste. In the 1990s they used to put the PURPOSE for their ingredients on the toothpaste box. So, they had a list of about six ingredients in one column, and the purpose for each ingredient right across from it in another column. They stopped doing this. Now they just list the ingredients, and shockingly, GLUTAMATE is ingredient number seven. This is why I don't use toothpaste that frequently. Glutamate, Excitotoxin, is in my Health Food toothpaste. Terrible.

JPM Oral Hygiene AM Protocol™
Brush – toothpaste
Floss
Mouth Rinse – 1T H_2O_2 30-60sec
Mouth Wash – 20% vodka gargle & rinse 10-15sec

Throughout the day and after eating:
Brush – no toothpaste
Floss
Mouth Wash – 20% alcohol gargle and rinse

JPM Oral Hygiene BB Protocol™
Before Bed same as AM

Hard/Firm toothbrush if my tongue feels a gritty film anywhere. Scaling tool once a week on anterior lowers (minerals in my saliva tend to precipitate on the backs of my lower teeth). And I use one of those long Oral B-60 toothbrushes to clean my tongue AM and PM. A lot of people neglect their tongue hygiene.

If you don't already own one, a Must-Have is an electric toothbrush.   Hand brushing simply can't compare to the fast vibrating movement of an electric toothbrush.   Philips Sonicare $35, works great. I keep one in my car. (No that's not weird.)

I am not as fortunate as my brother in that I still go to get my teeth cleaned every 6-12 months, but my hygienist and dentist always remark at how good my gums look, and how clean my teeth are. Apparently, a lot of teenagers have poor gum health and oral hygiene. Soft drinks! It's liquid sugar. The NCD considers soda pops as poisons, especially acidic colas. They're Anti-Nutrition. Health destroying.

Recall from the ABC NCD that – No amount of good can counter the bad you expose yourself to daily. You've got to eliminate the bad. In the old days, I can remember coke being used to remove the corroded-metal buildup from the posts of a car battery. And it worked good. Think about what it's doing to your teeth and gums.

As a final note, my next project is to discontinue using 3% topical hydrogen peroxide from the body-care aisle, and order 35% food-grade hydrogen peroxide from www.purehealthdiscounts.net. Then, just dilute it to about 3% by adding 1.5 ounces of the 35% H_2O_2 to the worcester bottle and then filling it to the top with water. See *Nontoxic Teeth Whitening and Dental Hygiene System*

And as another word of caution regarding the use of hydrogen peroxide as a mouth rinse.

IT'S NOT RECOMMENDED IF YOU HAVE METAL FILLINGS.

The H_2O_2 will, on a small scale, dissolve the metal, and those metal atoms can then be absorbed into your bloodstream via the capillary beds underneath your tongue, causing you to auto-intoxicate yourself over time. But if you have metal fillings in your mouth, your saliva is doing the same thing to a lesser degree 24-hours-a-day 7-days-a-week. If it was me, I would still do the hydrogen-peroxide mouth rinse AM and PM, as the benefits of having attached gingiva and healthy gums outweighs the risk of trace amounts of metal dissolving, getting into the bloodstream, and traveling to various locations within the body. Best advice is to have them removed and redone with composite, PLASTIC!

As a benefit to using the H_2O_2 mouth rinse AM and PM, you'll have nice white teeth! Peroxide is the active ingredient in most teeth whiteners.

Hope You Enjoyed This.

Jumper Publications & Media
Your First Choice for Selfcare

Once you've set up these two oral hygiene protocols and begin to see the benefits for yourself, why not hit the website and purchase a copy for a friend or family member, boss, coworker or your employees. For $30 you could purchase 10 copies and hand them out as "thank-you" tokens to people you know. Remember, it's fully copyrighted ISBN 978-1502489142 so making copies and free distribution is illegal – and bad Karma!

Chapter Endnote
The dictionary lists "drinking water" as a two word noun, water fit for drinking. However, I have hyphenated it in the chapters that follow to avoid reading it as "drinking" the verb and "water" the noun. If you read it as a unit "drinking-water" the sentences flow nicely.

PREVIEW
from the
ABC Water and the Number Crunch Diet

As you know, the recipes for the NCD are being published under the titles, *12 Changes a Year* – the companion guide to the Number Crunch Diet. It may take up to a year to get them written as it will comprise about three volumes. In the meantime, you can get your pH paper testing set up and determine your current alkaline stores. The recipes read like a book and include additional information that I've discovered about diet, lifestyle, health and selfcare. I look forward to seeing you over there!

To join my mission in providing people with safe, effective, affordable, selfcare protocols, send someone you know to www.abcwaterandthenumbercrunchdiet.com. Tell them to take the Quiz!! Thanks for your support! God Bless.

Jumper Publications & Media
from Advice to Results

I almost forgot! (again, not really) to tell you!

If you liked this shake recipe be sure to check out

TCY
12 Changes a Year
Vol 2

for the NCD ORANGE SHAKE!
It makes 9, and I often repeat the recipe midweek.
And whey protein – but not from powder.

BUY THE BOOK!!
IT'S GOOD STUFF!

FOLLOW-UP

You know, I've never liked the idea of brushing with baking soda because I've had in my mind all these years a picture of my dad brushing his teeth with the white-and-blue box of Arm & Hammer baking soda, and I assumed it was the one from the cleaning products aisle, which has contaminants and is too abrasive.

So, that glutamate in my toothpaste, and the fact that something in me, my Divine Intelligence, is telling me it's not good, has led me to rethink the baking soda for brushing.

Well, here's what you do. Buy baking soda in the BAKING aisle at a good-quality supermarket, I buy mine at Trader Joe's Market and it's USP, United States Pharmacopeia grade, the highest grade you can buy. To a 16oz glass jar, add the entire contents of the baking soda, use it to brush your teeth. Just wet the bristles and touch the powder, brush for two minutes, works great. Just the right amount of abrasion, not too rough not too mild. The food-grade USP baking soda in the baking aisle is so finely ground it's like a light soft powder, Perfect. The baking soda also gives your body a slight amount of bicarbonate, sodium bicarbonate, for alkalinity. See *ABC Water and the Number Crunch Diet* for the significance of alkalinity to good health, energy, and being ailment free.

So the JPM Oral Hygiene Protocol™ becomes,

1. food-grade or USP-grade baking soda to brush
2. 3% topical or food-grade hydrogen peroxide for gum lines
3. 20% food-grade vodka to gargle

The hydrogen peroxide and the baking soda will whiten.

If you do buy the 35% hydrogen peroxide, dilute it to 6% instead of 3% for a super-powerful teeth whitener! However, if you just be consistent and do the hydrogen-peroxide mouth rinse protocol AM and PM every day, you won't need more whitener. The 3% twice a day works perfectly. Happy Hygiene!

CHAPTER 11

Food Grade

If you read my website or book covers you will hear me refer to a "journey", "Come Join Me On The Journey To Health with the NCD Recipes and Omega 3 Protocol."

Well, I am going to make the switch from topical hydrogen peroxide to food grade, and it's so easy that I think you'll go-for-it as well after reading this.

The web address is www.drclarkstore.com, if you've read ABC NCD then you are already familiar with this company. The site prides itself on PURITY, based on the research and numerous books published by Dr. Hulda Clark. She has passed away, but it should be noted that all the talk in the mainstream, on newsfeeds, by Dr. Oz guests, on radio talk shows, in newspapers, magazines, the warnings of contaminants, contamination, heavy metals, polluted body products, polluted kitchen products, et cetera, all began with this independent researcher.

Her main book, *The Cure For All Diseases*, was published in 1995, so it takes about 10-15 years to penetrate into the mainstream.

If you are following Jumper Publications, you can consider yourself 10-15 years ahead of the mainstream. JPM – information and discoveries ahead of its time. Congratulations on being proactive and a person who reads!

Type "Hydrogen Peroxy" in the search-box and you will see two sizes. Buy two of the 6oz size. I used to buy this a few years ago and it was an 8oz size, but I think sellers require a special license to ship larger volumes of 35% hydrogen peroxide. For a larger size, you can order from www.purehealthdiscounts.net/h2o2.htm. Just keep it mind that hydrogen peroxide will turn into water if left uncapped, or when it gets hot.

So this 6oz size is fine, and if you use your 20%-off coupon that they will send you once you give them your email address or place your first order, then the price drops from $9.99 to x0.8 = $7.99, plus tax, free shipping if you spend $150. The cost works out to about $1 per week for clean gum lines.

The website says it's 35% food grade hydrogen peroxide and water. Now, keep in mind that this product is TWELVE times more concentrated than the 3% topical hydrogen peroxide in the body-care aisle. So Be Careful. It's not going to hurt you if you get it on your skin, but you will want to keep your eyes protected from this, like how you would protect your eyes from everything, hairspray, pesticides, air freshener, cigarette smoke. Hopefully you aren't using any of those things.

I've been making my own food-grade hairspray and styling gel for more than ten years. I will be publishing how to make it, so stay tuned for that. It's excellent. If you leave it in your hair overnight it doesn't harm your scalp or leave a scent on your pillow. I make it in four different strengths. In fact, I have a ginormous case of 800 white smooth-top spray pumps, so maybe I'll sell it to anyone interested in FOOD GRADE HAIRSPRAY!

But for now, we are doing food-grade whitening and dental hygiene.

$$C_1V_1 = C_2V_2$$

That's the formula we are going to use to determine how much of the 35% we need in order to have 3%.

Concentration of #1 times Volume of #1 = Concentration of #2 times Volume of #2.

Plugging in the numbers we have,

35% times X = 3% times 16oz

We have 35%, we want 3%, and the bottle we are using is 16oz.

Solve for X.

35% x X = 3% x 16oz

Divide both sides by 35% gives us,

$$X = \frac{3\% \times 16oz}{35\%}$$

The percents cancel top and bottom, and we are left with ounces.

Crunching the numbers we have 3x16÷35= 1.37oz or 1.4oz.

In my senior year I consistently got 100% on all the algebra and calculus exams and Garth, the guy sitting across from me, would go-off-the-deep-end when he would get his exam back and it said 94% or 96% and he would reach over to see mine and it was always 100%. He hated that. So it makes sense that I created and authored the Number Crunch Diet™. Don't worry, as I walk you through it over and over, in progressions. You'll do fine!

The DrClarkStore hydrogen peroxide comes in a squeeze bottle with nozzle top, so just cut the tip and add 1.4 ounces to each of your four worcester 16oz bottles. Place the bottle on the scale, turn it on, add H_2O_2 until it says 1.4 ounces, repeat repeat repeat.

The 6oz 35% H_2O_2 divided by 4 bottles is exactly 1.5 ounces, so you can add 1.5 ounces to each bottle, or do 1.4oz and add a couple of drops to each bottle at the end from the little bit left over.

Just for the record, using 1.5oz of the 35% and the 16oz bottle means that our final hydrogen peroxide will be 3.28% or 3.3%.

Fill your four worcester bottles up to the top, to the brim, to the level of the rim, with drinking-water, place the cap on and tighten it. This way, there should be zero air inside, or maybe just a tiny small bubble if you invert the bottle upside down. You don't need to mix it, but you can invert the bottle just to see if you have any air inside. A small air bubble is not a problem. The cap is perfect for making an airtight seal so no air will be getting inside as they sit on the shelf during the next few months while you use them up.

Now, take the second 6oz bottle of 35% H_2O_2 and repeat the same diluting steps as you just did, but using worcester bottles 5 6 7 8.

You now have a 4-month supply of your Secret Weapon. Do it AM and BB, twice a day, and you will have white teeth. And CLEAN gum lines. That's the most important reason for doing this.

If you've ever gotten your teeth cleaned, you no doubt have been instructed by your dental hygienist as to the correct way to brush your teeth. They say to angle the brush at 45 degrees and wiggle it so that the bristles of the brush clean the gum lines.

Well, that takes forever.

Plus, it's nowhere near as effective as using the hydrogen peroxide to flood the gum lines and to go underneath the gum, and between the teeth and underneath the gum. 360° gum-line cleaning.

Word to the Wise. SUGAR is evil. And LIQUID SUGAR is satan himself. It seeps into the pores of the teeth, under the gums, between the teeth, everywhere, and your tooth brushing is missing a lot of all those areas. Hence, every person I've ever worked with or met has a tooth filling, except my brother, 62 years old, and he will most likely live his entire life to 98 or beyond without a single cavity, tooth filling, or going to the dentist. Read my blog post about a 98-year-old relative who never saw a doctor her whole life.

My brother's also not someone who eats candy, sodas, chocolate, or sweets, and this helps.

Sugar also includes good sugar, like pineapple, grapes, oranges, and strawberries.   TEETH and SUGAR are not compatible. Unrefined sugar is different. The raw unfiltered honey used in the NCD Flaxseed Honey Shake™ contains propolis, which has antibacterial properties. But only in RAW honey, not liquid honey.

I would be lost without hydrogen peroxide, as I do eat fruit and some sweets. People who don't eat sugar tend to have perfect teeth, even with mediocre dental hygiene.

Storing your bottles of 3% H_2O_2. I store mine in the refrigerator, just because, but you can store them at room temperature, just keep in mind that if your room temperature is getting hot, your hydrogen peroxide may degrade some, or it may not have the same bubbling power on your last "swig" of the bottle that it had on the first swig.

Also, when you take your swig, open it, take your swig, close it. That cap should be off and back on in <10 seconds. Don't stand there swirling with the cap off.

Backwash. Now many of you may be thinking, "I'm not buying 8 worcester bottles at the supermarket and scrubbing the labels off."

Trust me, this is the perfect bottle, for these reasons.
1. It's 16oz so it will last one month, ½ an ounce per swig.
2. 8 bottles keeps you from running out, if you run out you won't do it.
3. Amber. To protect it from light, like the brown plastic bottles.
Note: the 6oz 35% H_2O_2 from drclarkstore comes in a translucent plastic bottle, but it's made on-demand, then it's placed in a box.
4. Airtight – the cap is long and threaded so it makes an airtight seal, and it's user-friendly, you tighten it and you're done, you don't have to "double-check" to see if it's on tight.
5. Leakproof – I take a bottle with me when I travel and it stays leakproof upside down.

6. SMALL MOUTH OPENING – this is key. If the opening is too wide, you'll take a swig and then you'll "backwash" some of it back into the container because you have too much in your mouth. This will degrade your peroxide. The worcester bottle is perfect.
7. Glass – Nontoxic. When plastics get hot, they leach phthalates.
8. Less Garbage – in four months, you will discard two small 6oz plastic bottles from drclarkstore. If you purchase 16oz brown plastic bottles of hydrogen peroxide from the drugstore, you will be discarding eight of these 16oz bottles every four months, 24 a year.

If you don't want anyone to see the words "Lea & Perrins" on the upper glass area of your bottle, (which you can't really notice unless you hold it in your hand), you can purchase 16oz glass amber bottles from SKS or C&P , see *ABC Water and the Number Crunch Diet*, Chapter 7, "Glass Food Containers".

Also see Chapter 6, why you should become a "Plastiphobe".

You can rinse your mouth with water after the H_2O_2, but I follow it with the 20% vodka rinse. Perfect.

Word to the Wise. I use the 20% vodka-alcohol mouthwash as a general oral sanitizer and like I said, to rinse out the hydrogen peroxide. But as a general rule, I don't "need" mouthwash. You shouldn't "need" mouthwash.   But many people do need mouthwash, because they have decay going on in their mouths. Halitosis is sooooo offensive, and yet those people haven't purchased this booklet, and they need to.

If you want to do something win-win, buy 50 copies of this booklet and just hand them out to people you come in contact with, clerks, delivery people, coworkers, friends, family. Just tell them that you like the system so much that you bought 50 copies, and hand them out as "thank-yous".

Thank you!

CHAPTER 12

JPM Whitener™

Isn't this fantastic! We have all FOOD GRADE products.

1. The 40% vodka diluted 50/50 to 20% for mouth washing.

2. The baking-aisle baking soda, or USP grade, for brushing.

3. The 3% food-grade hydrogen-peroxide rinse for gum lines.

And now the whitener.

We are going to make three strengths so that if you have a lot of discoloration you can use the Level 4, if you have moderate discoloration you can use Level 3, and for mild discoloration, use Level 2.

JPM Whitener Levels™
Level 1 = 3%   Daily Use AM & BB – maintenance protocol
Level 2 = 4%   Mild Whitening Action
Level 3 = 5%   Moderate Whitening Action
Level 4 = 6%   High Whitening Action

We won't go any higher than 6% strength H_2O_2 as 8 and 10% is too strong. If you get some of the 35% on your finger, it will turn it white a little. No biggie. It doesn't hurt. But it's just such a good WHITENER it will make your skin white upon contact!

Now keep in mind, if your teeth are stained dark yellow from decades of coffee or red wine, it is going to take you six months to get to the point where you can just do the 3% twice a day. Even those expensive whitening treatments can only do so much. So be realistic, and patient, and consistent. And try to give up the coffee and red wine, or at least not as strong.

If you drink espressos, those home espresso machines were all-the-rage a few years ago, well, you might as well not even bother doing this. You're just going to whiten with the peroxide, and then darken with the espresso, then white with the peroxide, then darken, whiten darken whiten darken, and in six months be nowhere.

No amount of good can counter the bad you expose yourself to daily. You have to eliminate the bad.™

Read that once more for me.

Those two lines are so key.

The *ABC Water and the Number Crunch Diet* has dozens of those lines. Those keys.

The next part after those two lines goes:

Sometimes all you need to do to get well is to eliminate the bad.™

People obsess with taking products and supplements and this, that, and the other. If they would just cut out the bad.

But the trick is – You Have To Know What The Bad Is.™

If you bought this, then you are already on the Journey.

CHEMICALS are worse than BIOLOGICALS™

Well, you say, "I don't agree, what about SARS, H1N1, Ebola?"

To that I say this.

First, your tissues and body get torn up and damaged with chemicals, THEN, the stage is set for the biologicals to enter.

IF YOU STAY HARMFUL CHEMICAL FREE, THE BUGS CAN'T GET AT YOU.™

It's more than just being immune compromised. By becoming free of chemical exposure, drugstore toothpaste, mouthwash, absorbed under the tongue, deodorant, absorbed under the arm, shampoo and conditioners, absorbed into the scalp, hairspray, I used to absorb that one into my lungs when I came behind my mother when she was in the bathroom putting up her hair, if you can become free from chemical exposures, your body will be resistant to microorganisms. Read the ingredients in drugstore lotion.

And let's not forget air pollution, vehicle exhaust, workplace odors, and natural gas refinery and other industrial plants off-gassing and chemically cleaning their exhaust stacks.

And the food you're eating, the chemical preservatives, flavorings, stabilizers, color retainers, and we already discussed the isopropyl-alcohol trace residues.

You'll never get away from them, but you need to do all that you can to limit your total exposure. The system I've laid out may seem like a fair amount of work, but it's a one-time setup for a lifetime of assurance. With enough assurance, you won't feel you need insurance.

CHEMICALS TEAR UP YOUR TISSUES™

Nearly every pathologic tissue biopsy contains one kind of metal or another, nickel, aluminum, lead, cadmium, more aluminum.

It's the which came first, The Chicken or The Egg? Most times, it's the chemicals first, then the pathogens second.

So, for our 3% H_2O_2 we used 1.5oz of the 35% per 16oz bottle, times 8 bottles. For the 4%, we will use 1.8oz per 6 bottles, and add the remainder to the 7th bottle and filling the 7th bottle halfway only, with water. For 5% peroxide, add 2.3oz of the 35% to 5 worcester bottles and fill them to the top while adding the remainder to the 6th worcester bottle and filling it 1/4th of the way up. And for 6%, add 2.7oz of the 35% to 4 worcester bottles and add the remainder to the 5th bottle filling it 1/3rd of the way up.

Strength	# of full bottles	35% ounces	35% grams	35% remainder
Level 1 – 3%	8	1.5	39g	
Level 2 – 4%	6	1.8	52g	halfway
Level 3 – 5%	5	2.3	65g	1/4th way
Level 4 – 6%	4	2.7	78g	1/3rd way

The 3% is really 3.28% and the 4% is 3.94%, the 5% is 5.03%, and the 6% is 5.91%, it doesn't have to be EXACTLY 3% 4% 5% 6%. If you want exactly 3.0% 4.0% 5.0% 6.0%, use 39g 52g 65g and 78g respectively (see the 35% grams column).

The NCD readers are familiar with the rule. Measure using a scale and not with measuring cups and measuring spoons, because scale measuring is more accurate with fewer dishes to wash.

Measure by Weight & Crunch in Calories™

Get the book, really. It's excellent.

It's a synergy of nearly 100 books that I've read in the past 14 years, more than 100 if I include college and university textbooks. Plus my ten years in the arts, teaching, performing, and choreographing, in ballet, tap, and jazz, and my bartending and waitering background, my grocery store experience, the cook/broilerman experience at the steakhouse. And the best one so far – Author of Selfcare Strategies!

No big company's going to tell you what I reveal in the book.

So there you have it. Use whichever level you need. Then when you get them to the shade you're satisfied with, then switch to the 3% twice a day maintenance protocol.

If you do these four things,

Food Grade teeth brushing
Food Grade gum line cleaning
Food Grade mouth washing
Food Grade teeth whitening

you won't need anything else.

Except the Sonic electric toothbrush for that fast vibrating action.

A long Oral B-60 toothbrush for tongue cleaning, tongue hygiene.

A hard/firm toothbrush for any areas where you feel a film or grit.

The scaling tool if needed occasionally or weekly.

And Dental Floss.

I used to use "Glide Tape" by Crest, as the floss is wider, like tape. But sometimes I would end up coming down hard on the gum tissue, so I stopped using it.

That's when I switched to the "Stretchy Tape" floss, Reach brand, "Total Care" or "Ultraclean". You can stretch it thin to get past the contact point, then floss up-and-down. If you hit your gum tissue, no biggie, as it won't hurt, and it doesn't turn your fingers blue either!

If you can find unflavored stretchy-tape floss, send an email and let me know. Those guys, they flavor everything. Chemical Flavors! I'll be adding onto this booklet with a commentary regarding fluoride. Wouldn't you like to know if it's something you should be doing, or should not be doing? Email me for the update.

CHAPTER 13

Fluoride Commentary

Hi again! Lucky for you, this edition contains the fluoride commentary. That's putting it lightly. If you've read the book, *The Fluoride Deception* by Christopher Bryson, you will know that the "fluoride commentary" that I am about to present is centered on a 50-year-long lie. Terrible.

If you check the reviews for *The Fluoride Deception* on Amazon, you will see 72 five-star reviews out of 77 total reviews. That's 94% five-star reviews. One person wrote a one-star review, calling it a conspiracy that would require the cooperation of tens-of-thousands of healthcare workers over decades.

Well, that's not hard to do.

You do what you're told to keep your job, right? If you object, you're blacklisted, and targeted for removal. This is the real world.

This one-star reviewer goes on to say that, "None of the author's claims hold up." The book contains 100 pages of endnotes. This is where "spin" and liars need to be called out and rebuffed, rebuked, and rebutted. Or, just leave them alone, to suffer in their delusional ignorance. Don't waste your energy with these people. The truth is not for them.

I read the 100 pages of endnotes and it was very dry, as it's lots and lots and lots of cited and documented material to back up the 250 pages of the main part of the book.

This one-star reviewer goes on to say that, "Community water fluoridation has been providing safe and effective protection from dental decay for years." Who is this person citing? Where is the evidence to prove it? Clearly, he's working for someone, or just another mind-controlled drone repeating what he heard on TV.

His is the only one-star review. The other 72 people that gave five-star reviews are obviously in the majority, 72 to 1.

I kept an open mind about fluoride, after all, I want to have hard strong teeth, as do most people. But, fluoride is not the answer. Industrial fluoride is a toxic chemical, even in small ppm amounts.

It's a fifty-year drama that goes back to World War II. The military and government needed fluoride to produce uranium for bombs, and they didn't need the public thinking that it was toxic.

Industry was in the same boat. Aluminum manufacturing was a booming business and the companies didn't want to be hindered with pollution-control laws or be spending millions of their profit dollars on equipment to make their plant operations cleaner. We're providing jobs, so just leave us alone. Or better yet, support us.

I am not going to get into all the details of the decades of fighting between the truthers and the liars, but I will highlight some things that I think you should know.

1. Prior to 1938, everyone, including the government and courts, agreed that fluoride was a poison. There was no pro-fluoride literature. It was like mercury or radium. But then, a deal was made in the backroom, or today, it would be done on the golf course. Gradually, the "machine", that grinds through all the levels of the pyramid, the structure of our society, that pyramid hierarchy, that top-down policy-making machine, changed everything. People began to hear that fluoride was good for your teeth.

2.   The key player who changed fluoride's image was also responsible for saying that, "lead in gasoline is safe". He spent his entire career claiming that the lead in gasoline was safe, even after it was unanimously proven unsafe and removed from gasoline. So right there, that tells me, this person, Dr. Xxxx, was a liar.

3. The book cites several noble scientists fired for stating the facts. Facts that industry didn't want to hear. This still goes on today. Or, if your conclusions don't support what we want, we pull your funding.

So there's nothing new under the sun. Life is a battle between good and evil, truth and lies, greedy corporations wanting to keep massive profits versus the slave employees getting a token for their back-breaking work. Oh, and one more, age, we love young and beautiful, and we want to toss anyone over fifty to the curb. We admire strong and detest weak. We respect those with wealth, and loathe those who are poor. It's the world we live in. Nothing new under the sun. It just is. Don't judge it. Just see it. So you can come to understand it better.

4. Eventually, pollution-control laws were passed in the 1970s, so clearly, the prior decades were in violation. Time eventually proved the truth.

5. But fluoride still goes untouched. Once the machine gave it the new image of being good for your teeth, no one challenged it. Well, people did, even doctors and dentists, but they were always silenced, removed, intimidated, or they simply wore out and threw-in-the-towel. Again, this still goes on today. If the people fight a new law and win, the opposition just resubmits it two-years later when the people have disbanded and things have quieted down.

So, fluoride is written in the history books as good for your teeth and "our history books record the facts". They record our greatest achievements and show why our nation is the world leader, so don't say anything negative about fluoride. Luckily, we are still free to read, think, and evaluate for ourselves.

CHAPTER 14

Strong Teeth Strategy

Those three pages barely touch the whole story of fluoride. But let's move on to the logic, analysis, and action plan.

Number one, hard bones aren't necessarily good. It's called "brittle bones". Your bones are so hard they just break, like how you would snap a stick of chalk in half. You don't want 'hard' bones.

Your bones need to be slightly bendable.

So number one, stop thinking that harder is better. It's not.

Keep in mind, that fluoridated water is full-body fluoridation. That means your bones are getting harder.

Full-body fluoridation is different from topical fluoridation.

Placing some topical fluoride on your teeth is not necessarily bad. However, drinking fluoridated water is bad.

So, number two, topical and systemic are two different things.

Topical fluoride treatments performed once a year or once every six months might not be a bad thing. Systemic fluoride taken daily via fluoridated drinking-water is bad. A lot of the people in the book that worked with fluoride had arthritis, big knuckles, and bony growths. Their bodies were taking that excess fluoride and putting it into their bones. And it was also in their tissues. Tissues are supposed to be soft squishy organs, not hard and tough.

So, do we need fluoride?

Well, your bones and teeth do contain some fluoride. Notice I said "some", a little, not that much. When you think of bones, you should be thinking CALCIUM. Milk. Cheese. Yogurt. The NCD recommends you wean yourself back on to milk, Chapter 57.

We get plenty of fluoride already. We don't need to supplement with fluoride. That means, we don't need to be adding it to the water.

#1 We don't need more.
#2 We don't need it systemically.

And #3, it's not healthy fluoride, like from mountain runoff water. It's industrial fluoride. So, #3, even if we did need more fluoride, supplementing with industrial fluoride is not the way to get it.

I recently asked an employee working in the supplement department at Lassen's, my local healthfood store, if she had any fluoride. There are hundreds of supplement products on their shelves. She thought about it, and then said, "no". They don't sell fluoride at the healthfood store. The bone supplements are always the same, calcium, magnesium, and vitamin D. You will never find fluoride listed as part of a bone mineral supplement, or on a multivitamin mineral supplement. But the government insists that it's a needed supplement and so they add it to the water. Agencies are not always correct. Surely, you must be aware of this. Governments are also very prideful, so they rarely retract a claim. They need to "save face" so as to maintain the confidence of the people. Recognizing this will help you to see more clearly, discern.

So, #1, we don't need very much fluoride for our bones, so we don't need to "seek it out" and actively try to get it. We get plenty.

And #2, we don't need to be supplementing it systemically, via the drinking-water.

And #3, if we did need to supplement, supplementing with industrial fluoride is like buying your mineral supplement from a concrete quarry. It's not clean.

And #4, fluoride is not a part of any bone-supplement products.

Now, they do sell fluoride supplements and give them to children. For a brief period I bought the one-gallon jugs of fluoridated water in the baby aisle at the supermarket. But I quickly sensed that this was not wise, and I tossed the second gallon down the drain.

So, #5, if you check with your Inner Divine Intelligence, you will know that it doesn't need any additional fluoride. It gets lots already. What it does need is, omega-3 fat, fish-oil fat, plant-color nutrients, alkalinity, and on and on. See the *Number Crunch Diet*. If you ask your Inner Divine, it knows, more fluoride is not needed.

Animals are extremely smart when it comes to knowing what they need. A cat can sense within a few seconds whether the food is something it should eat or not. They understand nutrition.

And, #6, we don't want hard hard bones. Note, excess fluoride can accumulate in the lens of the eyes. Cataracts anyone?

Topical fluoride treatments that your dental hygienist does are probably okay, but I don't do them. The water that's used to water the crops likely has fluoride in it, so the fruits and vegetables contain fluoride. And the livestock are likely drinking water that has fluoride in it, so the meat that we buy at the supermarket contains some fluoride. I don't need more.

What we do need, is to be sure we are getting GOOD, and not getting BAD. That is a much better plan.

So, rather than give your kids fluoride supplements, stop buying fruit juices and soft drinks and start feeding them milk as their only beverage. And not chocolate milk. White milk. If they are growing and have normal body fat, then feed them whole milk, if they are a bit overweight, feed them 2% milk. It's the sugar beverages that's making them fat, by keeping their insulin spiked all the time. See ABC NCD and TCY.

Don't let your kids drink anything other than milk for their beverage. And they can have water. Unfluoridated.

No one, not even children, should be drinking fluoridated water.

If you want to give them fluoride treatments every six months during their formative years, fine. But, by the time they reach adult age, their teeth are formed, so supplementing with topical fluoride treatments is pointless. Even the government will say that fluoride supplementation is for the formative years.

Also, keep your children's teeth clean, or have them do it, but check to make sure they are cleaning their teeth. Food that sits on your gum lines or between your teeth is going to cause tooth decay. No amount of fluoride will protect you from bad oral hygiene.

So, #1, **prevent demineralization of your teeth**, The Bad. This means, no sugar foods and NO SUGAR LIQUIDS. Also, no rotting food in your mouth. That means, no dirty gum lines and no food sitting between your teeth.

And #2, **support mineralization of your teeth**, The Good. Drink milk with its abundant naturally-occurring minerals, and vitamin D. Be sure to get outside and get vitamin D. You can't absorb minerals or nutrients without vitamin D. Tell your kids to go play outside, like kids did during the pre-technology pre-TV days. And have them use the *JPM Oral Hygiene Protocol* for clean gum lines, clean teeth, and clean spaces between teeth.

I worked with a woman who was relatively attractive and outgoing, but she had tan-colored teeth. I always thought it was from coffee stains. Then one day she told me that she has mottled teeth from fluoride and that no amount of whitening will change it.

One dentist I went to was very pro-fluoride. He was obsessed with "hard" teeth, but not understanding that, systemic fluoridation leads to hard tissues, boney growths, and overly-hard brittle bones.

He also said, "It makes your teeth brown, but it's worth it."

Honestly, with such an emphasis on having white teeth these days, I don't think anyone would want discolored teeth. In the 1970s and 80s, teeth whitening wasn't something anybody did. But in the 1990s teeth whitening exploded and spread like wildfire across the globe. And now, your employer, your friends, your family, everyone you meet, all expect you to have white teeth. You wouldn't wear a dingy yellowy-white blouse or shirt to work.

Your teeth color should look like white milk.

Fluoride's not the answer. The answer is in what you are holding in your hands. JPM – *Your First Source For Selfcare*

Chapter Endnote
You may have noticed that when there's a quotation within a sentence, that I place the comma on the outside of the quotation mark. Many writers and grammarians say you should place the comma inside the quotation. However, this gives the impression that the comma is part of the quotation. I keep my quotations "clean", and place the comma on the outside. Sorry grammarians.

Leave a Review

Without giving away the contents, "spoilers", recommend this publication and leave a review so that someone else might benefit from it too. Thank you.

www.amazon.com   Search: Nontoxic Teeth Whitening

Subscribe to my YouTube Channel
www.youtube.com   Search: Number Crunch Diet

Be sure to send me an email so I can periodically keep in touch with updates and new Selfcare Strategies – and discount offers on new items (yes, more than books!) (a simple and effective weight-loss device) (weightlifting "device" that I use EVERY time I work out) and don't forget the recipes! – TCY.

abcwaterandthenumbercrunchdiet@mail.com
Privacy – your email address will not be used for anything other than by Jumper Publications and Media.

Saliva vs Urine pH

Top Ten Reasons Why Saliva pH Is Worthless When Compared To Urine pH For Acid-Base Analysis

#10 Small Volume – small tiny volume samples don't represent the whole

#9 Difficult to Obtain – the procedure is to bring up saliva and swallow, 2x, then use the third one for the test, too hard to obtain

#8 Poor Reproducibility – when you retest your saliva sample, you will likely get a slightly different color (reading)

#7 Poor Accuracy – if you collect a second sample, it will likely give you a different reading than the first

#6 Bacterial Contamination – bacteria from your mouth will interfere with the test

#5 Food Contamination – food from your mouth will interfere with the test

#4 Spoon Contamination – the surface of the spoon that you collect it on is going to affect your small sample

#3 Viscosity – saliva is too thick and results in faded or dual colors of the test pad (or paper)

#2 Difficulty Reading – the color doesn't "lock in" so you can take a reading, it tends to change shades through a range

#1 Your Salivary Glands have ZERO to do with Acid-Base regulation. Try Kidneys.

Your kidneys are running your body's alkaline status.

And your alkaline status is the secret they don't want you to know.

JPM Oral Hygiene Protocol

This publication is the introduction to JPM. If you paid $2.99 for the kindle version or $4.99 for the paperback version, then you basically paid for the two protocols, the 20% vodka mouthwash, and the Secret Weapon, H_2O_2 gum-line cleaner. You will notice advertising for the other publications. Don't be upset. You got your $3-5 worth. The same cost as for a venti mocha latte, that's long since gone. The information in this publication will be with you for you to use for the rest of your life, every day.

So, why not take the ABC NCD Quiz!

The first half of the book is all about alkalinity. The secret aspect to your health no one, but a few, will talk about. However, no one covers the subject better and more comprehensively than in ABC Water™. The second half is the Number Crunch Diet™. No recipes, but lots of good sound information on diet. You will learn a lot, as no one discusses it the way I do. I brag a bit about the book, because it's really a great book. It's a compilation of nearly 100 books that I've read. But more of a Synergy, a new approach.

The recipes can be found in *12 Changes A Year* and you can see a sample on www.abcwaterandthenumbercrunchdiet.com

The title *Nontoxic Teeth Whitening and Dental Hygiene System* begins with the two chapters you just read, but includes a one-of-a-kind food-grade teeth whitening system, if you feel you need more whitening. It also includes a commentary on fluoride. Wouldn't you like to know if fluoride's something you should be doing, or something you shouldn't be doing?

So put your thinking cap on and let's start the Quiz!

It's good for you!

Pick the correct answers – There may be more than one

1. A urine pH of 5 is telling you
   a. about your blood pressure
   b. that you're tired
   c. about your alkaline reserves
   d. to see a doctor
   e. that you're healthy and fine

2. Urine pH testing is routinely performed by licensed
   a. social workers
   b. clinical laboratory scientists
   c. respiratory therapists
   d. fitness advisors
   e. nurses and doctors

3. The cost of one month of urine pH testing is _____ the cost of open heart surgery (CABG).
   a. 1/10
   b. 1/100
   c. 1/1000
   d. 1/10,000
   e. 1/100,000

4. The opposite of metabolic acid is dietary
   a. phosphates – found in meats and cola drinks
   b. bicarbonate – found in packaged foods
   c. caffeine – found in green tea
   d. bicarbonate – found in fruits and vegetables
   e. bicarbonate – found in oils and fats

5. Information can be of which types
   a. true
   b. incomplete

c. false

d. clouded

e. secret

6. "Natural Flavor" on a food label is
   a. natural flavor extracts from plants and fruit
   b. glutamates, MSG, altered salts
   c. chemicals that make you addicted to the product
   d. generally safe and good for me
   e. not something I need to worry about

7. During World War II, the people who failed to act early
   a. suffered
   b. died
   c. lost everything
   d. became victims
   e. made it through unscathed

8. Compensating means
   a. saving for retirement
   b. eating foods that lift your mood
   c. doing something to mask something
   d. brushing it out of your thoughts
   e. pleasing others and being a do-gooder
   f. all of the above

9. The reason(s) people are fat
   a. they're born that way
   b. they don't make their own meals
   c. hereditary – handed down from your parents
   d. my body just won't lose fat
   e. they don't see the numbers in what they're eating

10. The "Cheat Day" is
   a. a great way to get food cravings satisfied
   b. required to reset my fat-burning hormones
   c. a 2-8 step backwards day
   d. works well for most people long term
   e. is a popular "trick" that you should buy into

ANSWERS

1. A urine pH of 5 is telling you
   a. about your blood pressure – No, but there is a relationship
      (see Chapter 24)
   b. that you're tired – No, but there is a relationship (see Chapter
      20)
   c. about your alkaline reserves – YES! Get to know your
      alkaline status by reading this book.
   d. to see a doctor – No, but it can lead to that.
   e. that you're healthy and fine – One number tells you little, 35
      numbers a week tells you a lot. Get to know your urine pH.

2. Urine pH testing is routinely performed by licensed
   a. social workers – no
   b. clinical laboratory scientists – Yes, 99% of all urine testing is
      done by a CLS.
   c. respiratory therapists – no
   d. fitness advisors – no
   e. nurses and doctors – Doctors do perform urine tests in their
      offices, but they are not looking at urine pH with much depth.

3. The cost of one month of urine pH testing is _____ the cost of
   open heart surgery (CABG)(a bypass, "cabbage").
   a. 1/10 – no
   b. 1/100 – no
   c. 1/1000 – no
   d. 1/10,000 – Yes. You can test all of your urinations for about

$1 a month (see Chapter 11). A cabbage would run you at least $10,000.
e. 1/100,000 – no. But I believe the potential to save yourself $100,000 in medical treatments is very possible.

4. The opposite of metabolic acid is dietary
   a. phosphates – no, phosphates contribute to acidity
   b. bicarbonate – no, bicarbonate yes, but not from packaged foods
   c. caffeine – no, caffeine is a drug, most drugs are acidic
   d. bicarbonate found in fruits and vegetables – Yes!
   e. bicarbonate found in oils and fats – no, oils and fats are not sources of bicarbonate

5. Information can be of which types
   a. true – Yes, this is a bit what your life is all about. Finding the truth about things.
   b. incomplete – aka, partial truths or half truths, aka, "spin". Do you find your head spinning when you go for fancy medical treatments?
   c. false – lies, yes lies. Don't call them untruths. Lies are Lies. When people lie it's your job to call them on it. Otherwise, "ya got no backbone".
   d. clouded – blurry, muddied, confusion. I could write "scientifically" but I would just make you confused and half lost. How does that help you.
   e. secret – Now we're talking. When they say "buy this stock" you've got to be a moron to buy it. The payoffs and the winners are kept secret, shared through word of mouth.

6. "Natural Flavor" on a food label is
   a. natural flavor extracts from plants and fruit – Well, they would like you to think that, but that's far from reality.
   b. glutamates, MSG, altered salts – Yes, often this is the case.
   c. chemicals that make you addicted to the product – Yes

Absolutely
d. generally safe and good for me – don't buy that line
e. not something I need to worry about – you make your own choices in life

7. During World War II, the people that failed to act early
Referring to this is grim and bleak. But there are people suffering and dying every day because they failed to act early. You could say that WWII is still happening all around us in the United States of America today. My book can help you not to fall victim to this death and suffering.   So that you make it through your life, unscathed.

8. Compensating means
a. saving for retirement – no, but I have seen people who are just a little too attached to their portfolios, compensating?
b. eating foods that lift your mood – no, but food is commonly used to compensate
c. doing something to mask something – Ah-Ha, Yes.
d. brushing it out of your thoughts – no. It's okay and healthy to let go of thoughts, just be sure you're not avoiding your issues.
e. people pleasing – reward seekers may be compensating
f. all of the above – no, just C. Go back and read C again.

9. The reason(s) people are fat
a. they're born that way – don't give me that
b. they don't make their own meals – Bingo! This is key.
c. heredity – your fat jeans are because of your fat genes – no I don't think so
d. my body just won't lose fat – I hear you. There is not a lot of good help out there. Luckily, you've found the right place.
e. they don't see the numbers in what they're eating – Yes. And person D above just needs to look at food mathematically (and read the book).

10. The "Cheat Day" is
   a. a great way to get food cravings satisfied – Wrong. I'm a testimony of getting rid of food cravings. See Chapter 38, 39, 40, 41.
   b. required to reset my fat-burning hormones – Wrong. If you get your macros right, your hormones will cooperate just fine.
   c. a 2-8 step backwards day – On page 84 of *The Four Hour Body* the person states that he gains 4.4 lbs on his cheat day. Then he loses it. Can you say "moody"?
   d. works well for most people long term – After reading dozens of diet books, I could not find one that worked long term, so I made my own. It's called the Number Crunch Diet.
   e. a popular "trick" that you should buy into – The Number Crunch Diet isn't about cheating. Although it's full of useful "tricks" that I came up with and use daily.

You'll be miles ahead of the average person after a while.

FREE REPORT #1

JPM Hand Sanitizer™

So let's take this nontoxic thing a step further. If you heard the news about "triclosan", the chemical that they added to soap to make it "Anti-Bacterial Soap", well, that was in the 1990s and 2000s, and now in 2014 the mainstream media is reporting that Triclosan is cancer causing, liver damaging, and all the rest.

I never bought into it. I knew that it would just wipe out your normal skin flora and then the strong bugs would take over and populate. Your normal bacteria is harmless. There are two categories of bacteria, pathogenic, disease or infection causing, and non-pathogenic, harmless. If you remove the harmless bacteria, then the bad bacteria take over. Your good bacteria is keeping the bad bacteria from getting a foothold. As a microbiologist, I knew this. Sadly, the masses of people ran out and began buying up anti-bacterial soap and anti-bacterial sanitizer like it was the cure-all.

So, you can put Triclosan over in the category with the margarine and plastic bottled water. Another failed idea made by man with the sole purpose of selling products to nondiscerning consumers.

My job is to protect my readers from this deception. I see right through that stuff, and you will see it too after a while, many of you already do. So trust me when I say, you need to take the next step of chemical removal from your life, and that means, Personal and Household Sanitizer.

Back to our 40% vodka again, our food-grade alcohol, this was the recommended sanitizer in *The Cure For All Diseases*. Dr. Clark tested 40% vodka on many types of germs, the worst germ being parasite EGGS. Parasite eggs are walled-off, like the spores of yeasts and molds, this wall protects the life-form from being killed. It's their survival mechanism. So you think you are cleared of the germ, and 3-4 weeks later you break out in a rash again. The eggs have hatched. Gross, I know. But it's a real thing, especially for pet owners, those who swim outdoors, and areas with lots of birds.

Vodka kills those eggs. It is the only effective food-grade germ and microorganism killer for all categories of germs, including the designer germs, the genetically modified germs, e.g., MRSA, methicillin-resistant *Staphylococcus aureus*, the bacteria that is so aggressive that it doubles in size every 48-72 hours, and if it goes from your skin into your bloodstream, you're dead, unless you get to a hospital and have them give you IV vancomycin.

I visited a colleague CLS friend that I worked with and she had MRSA on her back. It drilled a hole and was making its way to her spinal column. Her doctor dropped-the-ball, and she took control of her treatment and saved her own life. She was on death's door when I saw her and she knew it. It was a close call, because MRSA moves fast, like I said, the bump or wound doesn't look like it's doing anything and then 72 hours later it doubles in size. If you ever see that happen, think MRSA, and get to a doctor for oral vancomycin. If it's already big, then go to a hospital ER and specifically ask for IV vancomycin. Many people die from MRSA, including a healthy teenager who picked it up in a locker room and didn't tell his parents that he had an infection, and the UPS worker who just thought it was a bump that would go away, and he didn't want to call in sick, and boom, dead a few days later. The designer GMO bugs can take down a healthy person, not just the elderly.

JPM Germs Defined™
1. Non-pathogenic, normal flora, the protective layer.
2. Pathogenic, disease causing, a strong body can usually kill it.
3. Designer bugs, engineered to kill, you need antibiotics to kill it.

So it's important to use a sanitizer, and one that's nontoxic, and that sanitizer is 40% vodka alcohol.

Go to your local drugstore and purchase a bunch of 2oz and 4oz spray bottles, with the fine-mist spray pump. Fill them with 40% vodka. The 2oz size is small enough to carry with you in your pocket or purse, and the 4oz size can be kept at your desk, in your car, in the bathroom, the kitchen, everywhere. Buy ten 4oz spray bottles and just put them all over your house. If you see it sitting there next to the door or on the counter, you will pick it up and use it. If you don't see it, you won't do it.

The 40% is strong enough to kill 99% of everything, including parasite eggs, mold spores, and genetically-modified bacteria.

You can dilute it 50/50 half-and-half with water and make 20% vodka and this is fine and adequate.

It even works at 10% strength, one-quarter 40% vodka and three-quarters water, but don't go any lower than 10%.

Personally, the cost is so little, that I never use 10% or 20% for sanitizing, I always use the 40%.

If you buy the 1.75 liter 40% vodka at Albertson's on sale for $8.99, then with tax it's about $10 for 1.75 liters. This is a lot of vodka for your money. You can fill ten of your 4oz spray-pump bottles and ten of your 2oz spray-pump bottles with this $10 bottle of 40% vodka. Those twenty spray-pump bottles would last you six months to a year. I use the 40% vodka to sanitize my wooden cutting board, my kitchen counters, the bathroom, to clean the mirrors, everywhere, and I probably only use one 1.75L bottle of vodka every five months. That works out to $2 per month for sanitizer. Effective, nontoxic, food-grade, sanitizer.

JPM Toothbrush Sanitizer™
After you brush your teeth and rinse your toothbrush, give the bristles one spray of the 40% vodka and let it air-dry. Perfect.

Free Report #1

Hand Sanitizer – Part 2

This next chapter will discuss more extensively the use of 40% vodka as an all-purpose personal and household sanitizer.

The drugstore 2oz and 4oz spray bottles are plastic. This is not ideal. I used plastic in the beginning, but two-years ago I switched them all to glass bottles. My local healthfood store actually sold 2oz and 4oz glass amber bottles with spray pumps. For $1.99 for the 2oz and $2.99 for the 4oz, I was able to replace all of my plastic spray bottles with glass for only $35. Then I went back and bought $20 more for extras. They will last a lifetime and you can use them in so many ways, or give them as gifts. If you go out for dinner with a friend, you can easily spend $35-40 and have nothing tangible to show for it. So spend the money and use glass sprayers.

If your local healthfood store doesn't have them, you can purchase Boston Round amber-glass bottles in 1oz 2oz 4oz 8oz sizes at www.containerandpackaging.com. Click on **Products** on the left, then click on **Glass Containers**, and then mouse over to **Glass Bottles** and click on that. Then click on the **Glass Boston Rounds** image, and there you have it, all sizes in glass amber bottles. You will need spray pumps. Click on the 4oz size and then click on **Fine Mist Sprayers** or **Smooth Pumps** and make a selection of your choice. Just be sure to match up the bottle-neck size with the spray-pump size, i.e., a 20-400 bottle neck will need a 20-400 spray pump. Call them if you need to confirm your order.

When you spend $50 or more you avoid the $10 small-order fee. So spend some time deciding and place a $50 order and fill your house with 2oz and 4oz spray bottles with 40% vodka.

You can feel comfortable knowing that all the sanitizing you do is nontoxic, chemical free, and not going to harm you, enter your skin, tissues, and build up in the organs. I highly recommend this.

Okay, so we spray our toothbrush after using it, we spray our wooden cutting board after washing it, we spray our kitchen counter before and after food prepping, and we spray our hands.

Hand Spraying Technique. Hold the spray bottle in your right hand, bring your four fingers and thumb of your left hand together, in the "chicken pecking" position, all five of your fingers touching and there is a golfball-sized empty space. Now, with your five fingernails together and facing you, spray your 40% vodka four times aiming it right into the nails. Now switch hands and do the same thing with the right, place all five fingers of your right hand together, facing you, and use the left hand to spray four times at the nails. Now, rub your two hands together on all sides, top of your hands, palms of your hands, between your fingers, between the thumb and index finger, interlock your right and left hand fingers and move them around a bit, and then move down to the wrist and get some vodka on your wrists, right and left. Your hands are now dry, sanitized, and clean. Total time, 10 seconds.

JPM Hand Sanitizing™
With the palm of your left hand facing you, bring your fingers and thumb together, point the sprayer of 40% vodka at your five fingernails and spray them four times, repeat with the other hand. Rub your hands together and spread the liquid all over your hands, fingers, and wrists, on all sides, ten seconds is good. That's it. You just sanitized your hands, but especially your nails.

It took me a while to come up with this technique, and it is perfect. The four sprays flood the nails, then as it begins to drip down your fingers a bit, you spread it all over your hands and wrists, and in ten seconds it's dry. Perfect. And it doesn't dry out my skin, not even a little bit, not even in the winter.

You can spray your toenails when you get out of the shower. I use it in place of deodorant, just three sprays under each arm, once a day, and never any odor, no bacteria. If you want to dry up a pimple, it works for that too. I had an oily sebaceous cyst on the back of my shoulder that was removed 25-years ago, but it comes back a little bit sometimes. However, as long as I give it a spray shot with the vodka once a day after my shower, it says flat and never develops a head.

The next section is a bit graphic and you can skip this and jump to the next chapter if you want. But I think it's excellent hygiene, and many people could benefit from it.

I stopped using bathroom paper and switched to using Kleenex facial tissue. Someone I know did this and I came to discover that Kleenex feels so soft on your butt area. Use the 2-ply Kleenex, the big boxes, and it's not going to cost you much more money than regular bathroom paper. So, use three Kleenex sheets per wipe. Then for a final clean, take three Kleenex sheets, spray them with the 40% vodka and do a sanitize of the area. You will be surprised by how much cleaner you really are if you do this.

If you keep these areas of your body clean, sanitized, people will notice that you are extra clean. Like a brand-new shirt, or brand-new carpet, you will just give the impression that you are clean from the top of your head to the tip of your toenails, and everywhere in between. Even in a professional work environment, there was at least one person a day that had some unpleasant smell, either halitosis, or just something slightly "not fresh" about them. Don't let that be you.

FREE REPORT #2

JPM Vodka Towelette™

Okay, we are not done sanitizing. In addition to the 2oz and 4oz 40% vodka glass spray-pump bottles for sanitizing, you should also use the JPM Vodka Towelettes™.

You have to make them. But it's not hard. Well, not hard, but a little bit of work. Just watch TV while you make them.

You will need a 32oz pump bottle, like a 32oz shampoo pump bottle, but don't use a shampoo bottle because the smell of the shampoo will never come out of the bottle no matter how much you rinse and clean it. Those shampoo chemicals and fragrances are permanently inside the plastic, so you will need to buy a brand-new container. I bought mine at www.sks-bottle.com, and if you've read *ABC Water and the Number Crunch Diet*, then you will recognize this site, as it's where we purchase glass food containers. If you order this 32oz pump bottle with your glass food containers and spend $250 then it's free shipping, otherwise you will have to pay shipping for this 32oz pump bottle.

Type **0012-35** into the search-box, then click on the **Pump Dispenser** image. You will see a 32oz plastic bottle with a hand pump, item 0012-35, six bottles with pumps for $11.76. This pump is perfect. It's user-friendly and it will last. You can use the other five bottles for something else, or give them to your friends and have them make the JPM Vodka Towelettes™ too!

So we have our 32oz pump dispenser for our 40% vodka sanitizer, now we need paper towels and snack sandwich bags.

Buy plain white paper towels, one-ply. I buy Scott Towel brand one-ply plain white paper towels, 11x11 inch sheets. Be sure the sheets are 11x11 inches.

Next, buy reclosable snack bags. They are like sandwich bags, but half the size, shorter, 6.5 inches x 3.25 inches (16.5cm x 8.25cm). Whereas a sandwich bag is square shaped, a snack bag is half the length and rectangular shaped. I buy mine at Smart and Final grocery and restaurant-supply store, 150 bags per box, but Walmart and all supermarkets sell them.

I like the First Street brand from S&F because the ziplock is good quality and easy to zip it closed, and the plastic is fairly thick. If the plastic is too thin, your towelettes will dry out sooner. If the ziplock doesn't seal or stay closed, then air will get inside and dry out your towelettes.

JPM Vodka Towelette™
1. 40% vodka with 32oz hand-pump dispenser
2. 11x11 plain white one-ply paper towels
3. reclosable snack bags, a good-quality brand
4. one-quart size reclosable food-storage bags

I also buy the one-quart food-storage reclosable bags at S&F, 100 per box, 7 inches x 8 inches, 17.8cm x 20.3cm, 0.94 liter, 1 quart.

You will place the snack bags of your vodka towelettes into the one-quart bag and zip it, "double bagged" for extended expiration.

Procedure
1. On a clean counter, pull 21 sheets of paper towel and by placing one hand on each side of the perforation, tear them apart. You will now have 21 sheets of 11x11 paper towel.
2. Fill your 32oz pump dispenser with 40% vodka and position it at three o'clock, to your right if you are right-handed.

3. Place 21 snack bags at ten o'clock.

4. Now, with the torn edges of the paper towel at east and west, fold the paper towel in half, south to north. Now, rotate it clockwise 90 degrees and fold it in half south to north again. And fold it in half south to north again.

So,

1. fold south to north (bottom to top)
2. rotate 90° clockwise
3. fold south to north
4. fold south to north again

You now have a paper towel that will fit perfectly inside your snack bag, the same size as your snack bag. Put the paper towel into your snack bag. Your paper towel has a folded edge and an open edge. Place it in the snack bag with the open edge at the bottom of the snack bag. The folded edge will be at the top of the snack bag next to the zip.

5. Now, hand pump four squirts of vodka into the snack bag. Four smooth pumps. Move the bag with each pump, i.e., one pump into the bag at the end, then one pump at almost the middle, then another pump past the middle, and the fourth pump at the other end.

Pump 1   Pump 2   Pump 3   Pump 4

So you move the bag as you pump the four pumps, getting vodka in all areas of the bag, and on the towelette.

Also, shoot your vodka at the top of the paper towel, and it will soak into the paper towel, which is what you want.

6. Lastly, place the bag on the counter and flatten it out to remove the air, then zip it by running your hand from right to left and squeezing out the air as you zip it closed.

Congratulations! You just made a Nontoxic Alcohol Towelette.

Now you can make 21 of these singles, and place 21 single towelettes in one of the one-quart bags. That's fine. I used to do this. But now I make triple-packs. Three paper towels in one snack bag, and then seven triple-pack snack bags into one one-quart bag.

So,
21 singles per one-quart bag, or
7 triple-packs per one-quart bag

With the singles, you open it, remove the towelette and throw the bag away and use the towelette and then throw the towelette away.

With the triple-packs, you remove one towelette, reseal it, and use the towelette and throw it away. Then you discard the bag with the third towelette. You throw away fewer bags with the triple-packs.

The singles are thinner and can easily be hidden in a pocket. You can pull it out before eating at the cafeteria or at a restaurant and sanitize your hands. The triple-pack is a bit bulkier, and would be good for keeping in your purse, or in a fanny pack, or a briefcase.

To make the triple-packs, fold your paper towel as before, then do it two more times, and stack them together and place them into your snack bag, open sides down, fold sides up. Then squirt 12 shots of vodka in, lay it on the counter, flatten out the air and zip it.

If the three paper towels aren't completely wet, don't worry, they will become saturated as the vodka spreads, the next morning the three towelettes will be completely wet and ready-to-use.

Surely you've all seen the hand-towelette dispenser at the supermarket and people take one or two and clean the handrail of the shopping cart. For me, there are no germs on that handrail that are going to harm me. However, the CHEMICALS in those towelettes are going to soak right into my skin and into my body.

People don't think.

People that don't read don't know.

These people are doing more harm to themselves than good by using those chemical towelettes. Those people that you see at the supermarket adamantly cleaning the rail of their cart and then their hands are the same people that ran out and bought anti-bacterial soap in the 1990s, and margarine in the 1980s. If you are reading this, then you are a well-informed person, and not fooled. You read. You think. You analyze. And you look at things from a more educated and informed angle. Kudos! You are my people! Say "hello" and drop me an email. I have more nontoxic chapters to come!, hairspray, styling gel, a stronger deodorant, and food-grade lotion.

Gifts, Christmas or Birthday. I often give this one-quart bag of vodka towelettes as a gift, the 21 singles or the 7 triple-packs. At first people aren't sure what it is. But I've printed labels on my computer and I label the one-quart bag with,

Hand Towelettes – ingredient, 40% food-grade grain alcohol (vodka).

The next time I talk to them they are telling me how much they liked them, how clean they felt, and how they liked the nonscent nonfragrance. Then they say, "Yeah, I've run out." Hint Hint. People love them, and I am certain you will too. Add this into your lifestyle and make your personal and household sanitizing nontoxic.

God Bless.

Shelf Life – the amount of time before they dry out
If you leave the single in your car on a hot day, it will dry out.
The single or triple-pack at room-temp will stay wet for 3-4 weeks.
Storing them in the one-quart bag in the refrigerator, six months.

If you don't have a computer and would like labels for the one-quart bag, email me and I can send you some labels through the post office. The label makes your bag of towelettes look like a "product" and a real gift. Your clean-living holistic friends will love them!

A friend of mine and I once visited a lady who was the ex-wife of the CEO of Carnation Milk Corporation. She was having a hard time living on $20,000 a month, as before the divorce she lived on $50,000 a month. So, for the wealthy out there, these nontoxic hand towelettes are perfect for you and your kids. I can mail you three bags of the singles every other month, that would be 21x3=63 towelettes, use one a day. Email me if you're interested. Many of you don't have time for "setup" or "making things" but have no problem with money. Hey, I can help you.

You can use a single towelette three times before throwing it away. I use one single a day. I use it to wipe my hands if I am eating lunch away from home, and then put it back in the bag, then use it once again later in the day, and put it back in the bag, and then use it a third time and toss it. Or you can use one triple-pack a day, or one triple-pack per two days. They really are a must-have for people who are out in public, at school, the workplace, airports, shopping malls, supermarkets, restaurants, everywhere.

Jumper Publications and Media
Your First Source For Selfcare

Chapter Endnote
Doesn't he know the difference between "bacteria" plural and "bacterium" singular? Of course. The "bacteria is" is referring to the "protective layer", the layer is. Your normal flora of protective bacteria number in the trillions, 100 trillion bacteria per person, outnumbering your human cells 10 to 1. I refer to them as one, your normal protective layer, and this paints a picture of "good". To use "bacterium" and "bacteria" gets too technical for most people, but just be aware of the two words. And good thing you're paying attention!

www.ingramcontent.com/pod-product-compliance
Lightning Source LLC
Chambersburg PA
CBHW060222290526
45789CB00003B/1377